FAST!
CHEAP!
DELICIOUS!
VEGAN RECIPES

Wholesome and Budget-Friendly Plant-Based Cuisine

MOH LIMS

Copyright©2023 Moh Lims

All right reserved

OTHER BOOKS BY THE AUTHORS

1. THE WILD GRIDDLE COOKBOOK
2. THE FLAME PROJECT
3. THE BARBECUE BIBLE PRO
4. THE MASTERING BARBECUE SAUCES
5. THE PELLET GRILL BIBLE
6. THE MICROWAVE EFFORTLESS COOKBOOK

TABLE OF CONTENT

INTRODUCTION

Welcome to the world of Fast, Cheap, and Delicious Vegan recipes! If you're looking for a delightful culinary adventure that won't break the bank and won't take hours to prepare, you've come to the right place.

In this collection, we've curated an array of mouthwatering dishes that prove vegan cuisine can be diverse, satisfying, and incredibly easy to whip up.

Our 20 carefully crafted recipes embrace the beauty of plant-based ingredients, showcasing a medley of vibrant fruits, vegetables, legumes, and whole grains.

From hearty soups to refreshing salads, from flavorful stir-fries to indulgent desserts, we've covered a range of dishes that will tantalize your taste buds and nourish your body with essential nutrients.

Whether you're a seasoned vegan or simply curious about incorporating more plant-based meals into your diet, our recipes are designed to please everyone. You'll discover that these creations not only taste incredible but also offer numerous health benefits.

Packed with fiber, vitamins, and minerals, these dishes support digestion, promote heart health, boost immunity, and provide sustained energy throughout your day.

So, roll up your sleeves, grab your apron, and get ready to embark on a culinary journey filled with flavor, goodness, and affordability. Whether you're cooking for yourself, your family, or hosting a gathering with friends, our Fast, Cheap, and Delicious Vegan recipes are sure to impress and leave a lasting impression on your taste buds and your health. Enjoy the process of cooking, and relish the joy of savoring each delectable bite.

Let's dive in and discover the magic of vegan cuisine together!

Recipe 1: Chickpea Salad

Ingredients:

- 1 can of chickpeas, drained and rinsed
- 1 cucumber, diced
- 1 red bell pepper, diced
- 1 small red onion, finely chopped
- 1 cup cherry tomatoes, halved
- Fresh parsley, chopped
- Juice of 1 lemon
- 2 tbsp olive oil
- Salt and pepper to taste

Instructions:

1. In a large bowl, combine the chickpeas, cucumber, bell pepper, onion, and cherry tomatoes.

2. In a separate small bowl, whisk together lemon juice, olive oil, salt, and pepper.

3. Pour the dressing over the salad and toss to combine.

4. Garnish with fresh parsley. Serve chilled.

Benefits:

This salad is rich in plant-based protein, fiber, and essential vitamins and minerals. It's excellent for digestion, supports heart health, and provides a boost of antioxidants.

Recipe 2: Lentil and Vegetable Stir-Fry

Ingredients:

- 1 cup dried green lentils, cooked
- 1 cup broccoli florets
- 1 cup sliced carrots
- 1 cup bell peppers, sliced
- 1 tbsp sesame oil
- 2 tbsp soy sauce
- 1 tbsp rice vinegar
- 2 cloves garlic, minced
- 1 tsp grated ginger

Instructions:

1. In a large skillet or wok, heat sesame oil over medium-high heat.
2. Add garlic and ginger, sauté for a minute.
3. Add the sliced carrots and cook for 2 minutes.
4. Add the bell peppers and broccoli, stir-fry for an additional 3-4 minutes until tender-crisp.

5. Stir in the cooked lentils, soy sauce, and rice vinegar. Cook for another 2 minutes, stirring frequently.

6. Serve over brown rice or quinoa.

Benefits:

This dish is packed with plant-based protein, iron, and fiber. It promotes healthy digestion, supports blood sugar balance, and is beneficial for weight management.

Recipe 3: Sweet Potato and Black Bean Quesadillas

Ingredients:

- 2 large sweet potatoes, cooked and mashed

- 1 can black beans, drained and rinsed

- 1 cup diced red bell pepper

- 1 cup diced red onion

- 1 tsp ground cumin

- 1 tsp chili powder

- 4 large whole wheat tortillas

- Vegan cheese (optional)

Instructions:

1. In a bowl, mix mashed sweet potatoes, black beans, red bell pepper, red onion, ground cumin, and chili powder.

2. Lay out one tortilla and spread a portion of the mixture on one-half of the tortilla.

3. If using vegan cheese, sprinkle some on top of the mixture.

4. Fold the tortilla in half, pressing down gently.

5. Cook the quesadilla on a non-stick pan over medium heat until both sides are golden brown and the filling is heated through.

6. Repeat with the remaining tortillas and filling.

7. Cut into wedges and serve with salsa or guacamole.

Benefits:

This dish is a great source of complex carbohydrates, protein, and essential nutrients like vitamin A, vitamin C, and potassium. It's filling, satisfying, and promotes overall health.

Recipe 4: One-Pot Coconut Curry

Ingredients:

- 1 cup diced potatoes
- 1 cup chopped carrots
- 1 cup chopped bell peppers
- 1 cup cauliflower florets
- 1 can coconut milk
- 2 tbsp red curry paste
- 1 tbsp soy sauce
- 1 tbsp vegetable oil
- Fresh cilantro for garnish
- Cooked rice or quinoa for serving

Instructions:

1. In a large pot, heat vegetable oil over medium heat.

2. Add the potatoes and carrots, sauté for 5 minutes.

3. Add the bell peppers and cauliflower, sauté for an additional 3 minutes.

4. Stir in the red curry paste and soy sauce, coating the vegetables evenly.

5. Pour in the coconut milk and bring to a simmer. Cook until the vegetables are tender.

6. Serve over cooked rice or quinoa, garnish with fresh cilantro.

Benefits:

This flavorful curry is rich in healthy fats from coconut milk and various vitamins and minerals from the vegetables. It supports immune function, aids digestion, and contributes to a balanced diet.

Recipe 5: Vegan Lentil Shepherd's Pie

Ingredients:

- 1 cup green lentils, cooked
- 1 cup diced carrots
- 1 cup peas (frozen or fresh)
- 1 cup corn kernels
- 1 onion, diced
- 2 cloves garlic, minced
- 1 tbsp tomato paste
- 2 cups vegetable broth
- 2 tbsp olive oil
- Mashed potatoes (prepared separately)

Instructions:

1. In a large skillet, heat olive oil over medium heat. Add onions and garlic, sauté until translucent.

2. Stir in the diced carrots, peas, and corn. Cook for 5 minutes.

3. Add the cooked lentils and tomato paste, mixing well.

4. Pour in the vegetable broth and simmer until the mixture thickens.

5. Preheat the oven to 375°F (190°C).

6. Transfer the lentil and vegetable mixture into a baking dish and spread an even layer of mashed potatoes on top.

7. Bake in the oven for 20-25 minutes or until the top is golden brown.

Benefits:

This hearty dish is an excellent source of plant-based protein, fiber, and various nutrients. It supports gut health, provides sustained energy, and is a delicious comfort food option.

Recipe 6: Zucchini Noodles with Avocado Pesto

Ingredients:

- 3 large zucchinis, spiralized or thinly sliced
- 1 ripe avocado
- 1 cup fresh basil leaves
- 1/4 cup pine nuts (or walnuts)
- 2 cloves garlic
- Juice of 1 lemon
- 2 tbsp nutritional yeast
- Salt and pepper to taste

Instructions:

1. In a food processor, combine avocado, basil, pine nuts, garlic, lemon juice, and nutritional yeast. Blend until smooth.
2. Season with salt and pepper to taste.
3. In a large pan, sauté the zucchini noodles for 2-3 minutes until slightly softened.
4. Toss the zucchini noodles with the avocado pesto until evenly coated.
5. Serve immediately, garnished with additional basil leaves if desired.

Benefits:

This light and flavorful dish are rich in healthy fats from avocado and pine nuts. It's a great option for those looking to cut down on carbohydrates, supports heart health, and provides essential vitamins and minerals.

Recipe 7: Black Bean and Quinoa Stuffed Bell Peppers

Ingredients:

- 4 large bell peppers, halved and seeds removed
- 1 cup cooked quinoa
- 1 can black beans, drained and rinsed
- 1 cup corn kernels
- 1 cup diced tomatoes
- 1 tsp ground cumin
- 1 tsp chili powder
- Salt and pepper to taste
- Vegan cheese (optional)

Instructions:

1. Preheat the oven to 375°F (190°C).

2. In a large bowl, combine cooked quinoa, black beans, corn, diced tomatoes, ground cumin, chili powder, salt, and pepper.

3. Stuff each halved bell pepper with the quinoa mixture.

4. Place the stuffed bell peppers on a baking dish and cover with foil.

5. Bake in the oven for 20-25 minutes or until the peppers are tender.

6. Optionally, add vegan cheese on top and bake for an additional 5 minutes until melted.

Benefits:

These stuffed bell peppers are a complete meal packed with protein, fiber, and essential nutrients. They support healthy digestion, provide sustained energy, and are an excellent option for a balanced diet.

Recipe 8: Vegan Thai Peanut Noodles

Ingredients:

- 8 oz rice noodles (or any other pasta)
- 1 cup broccoli florets
- 1 cup sliced bell peppers
- 1 cup shredded carrots
- 1/2 cup chopped scallions
- 1/4 cup creamy peanut butter
- 2 tbsp soy sauce

- 2 tbsp lime juice

- 1 tbsp maple syrup

- 1 tsp sesame oil

- Crushed peanuts and fresh cilantro for garnish

Instructions:

1. Cook the rice noodles according to package instructions. Drain and set aside.

2. In a small bowl, whisk together peanut butter, soy sauce, lime juice, maple syrup, and sesame oil until smooth.

3. In a large skillet, sauté broccoli, bell peppers, and shredded carrots for 3-4 minutes until slightly tender.

4. Add the cooked rice noodles and peanut sauce to the skillet, tossing to coat the noodles and vegetables evenly.

5. Garnish with crushed peanuts and fresh cilantro before serving.

Benefits:

This flavorful dish is rich in healthy fats from peanut butter, along with vitamins and minerals from the vegetables. It supports brain health, promotes satiety, and provides a delightful taste experience.

Recipe 9: Vegan Banana Oat Pancakes

Ingredients:

- 2 ripe bananas
- 1 cup rolled oats
- 1 cup plant-based milk (such as almond or soy milk)
- 1 tsp baking powder
- 1 tsp vanilla extract
- Pinch of salt
- Maple syrup and fresh fruit for topping

Instructions:

1. In a blender or food processor, blend the bananas, rolled oats, plant-based milk, baking powder, vanilla extract, and salt until smooth.

2. Heat a non-stick pan over medium heat.

3. Pour 1/4 cup of the pancake batter onto the pan for each pancake.

4. Cook until bubbles form on the surface, then flip and cook the other side until golden brown.

5. Serve with maple syrup and fresh fruit on top.

Benefits:

These pancakes are a nutritious breakfast option, providing fiber, potassium, and natural sweetness from bananas. They support heart health, provide sustained energy, and are a delightful morning treat.

Recipe 10: Vegan Lentil and Vegetable Soup

Ingredients:

- 1 cup dried red lentils
- 1 onion, diced
- 2 cloves garlic, minced
- 1 cup diced carrots
- 1 cup diced celery
- 1 cup diced tomatoes (canned or fresh)
- 6 cups vegetable broth
- 1 tsp ground cumin
- 1 tsp paprika
- Salt and pepper to taste
- Fresh parsley for garnish

Instructions:

1. Rinse the red lentils thoroughly and set aside.

2. In a large pot, sauté the onion and garlic until softened.

3. Add the diced carrots, celery, and tomatoes. Cook for an additional 5 minutes.

4. Pour in the vegetable broth and bring to a boil.

5. Stir in the red lentils, ground cumin, paprika, salt, and pepper.

6. Reduce the heat to low, cover the pot, and let the soup simmer for 20-25 minutes or until the lentils are tender.

7. Garnish with fresh parsley before serving.

Benefits:

This hearty and nutritious soup is rich in plant-based protein, fiber, and various vitamins and minerals. It supports immune function, aids digestion, and is perfect for cold days.

Recipe 11: Vegan Tofu and Vegetable Stir-Fry

Ingredients:

- 1 block of firm tofu, cubed

- 1 cup broccoli florets

- 1 cup sliced bell peppers

- 1 cup sliced mushrooms
- 1 cup snow peas
- 2 tbsp soy sauce
- 1 tbsp hoisin sauce
- 1 tbsp sesame oil
- 1 tsp grated ginger
- 2 cloves garlic, minced

Instructions:

1. In a large skillet or wok, heat sesame oil over medium-high heat.

2. Add minced garlic and grated ginger, sauté for a minute.

3. Add the cubed tofu and cook until lightly browned on all sides.

4. Stir in the broccoli, bell peppers, mushrooms, and snow peas. Cook for 4-5 minutes until vegetables are tender-crisp.

5. Mix in the soy sauce and hoisin sauce, tossing to coat the tofu and vegetables.

6. Serve over cooked rice or noodles.

Benefits:

This protein-packed stir-fry is a great source of calcium and iron from tofu, along with a variety of vitamins and minerals from the colorful vegetables. It supports bone health and overall vitality.

Recipe 12: Vegan Lentil Bolognese

Ingredients:

- 1 cup dried brown or green lentils, cooked
- 1 onion, diced
- 2 cloves garlic, minced
- 1 cup diced carrots
- 1 cup diced celery
- 1 can crushed tomatoes
- 1 tbsp tomato paste
- 1 tsp dried oregano
- 1 tsp dried basil
- Salt and pepper to taste
- Cooked spaghetti or your favorite pasta

Instructions:

1. In a large skillet, sauté onions and garlic until softened.
2. Add the diced carrots and celery, cooking for an additional 3-4 minutes.

3. Stir in the cooked lentils, crushed tomatoes, tomato paste, dried oregano, dried basil, salt, and pepper.

4. Let the sauce simmer for 15-20 minutes, allowing the flavors to meld.

5. Serve the Bolognese sauce over cooked pasta.

Benefits:

This hearty and satisfying dish is rich in protein, fiber, and antioxidants. It supports digestive health, contributes to balanced blood sugar levels, and makes for a comforting meal.

Recipe 13: Vegan Quinoa and Black Bean Burritos

Ingredients:

- 1 cup cooked quinoa
- 1 can black beans, drained and rinsed
- 1 cup diced tomatoes
- 1 cup diced avocado
- 1 cup shredded lettuce or spinach
- 1/4 cup chopped cilantro
- Juice of 1 lime
- 4 large whole wheat tortillas

Instructions:

1. In a large bowl, combine cooked quinoa, black beans, diced tomatoes, diced avocado, shredded lettuce or spinach, chopped cilantro, and lime juice.

2. Warm the tortillas on a dry skillet for a few seconds to make them pliable.

3. Spoon the quinoa and black bean mixture onto each tortilla, folding in the sides and rolling up tightly to form burritos.

4. Slice in half and serve.

Benefits:

These burritos are a complete meal, providing a balanced combination of protein, healthy fats, and fiber. They support heart health, provide satiety, and are perfect for on-the-go meals.

Recipe 14: Vegan Cauliflower Buffalo Wings

Ingredients:

- 1 head of cauliflower, cut into florets

- 1 cup almond flour

- 1 cup plant-based milk (such as almond or soy milk)

- 1 tsp garlic powder

- 1 tsp onion powder

- 1 cup buffalo sauce (store-bought or homemade)

Instructions:

1. Preheat the oven to 425°F (220°C). Line a baking sheet with parchment paper.

2. In a large bowl, whisk together almond flour, plant-based milk, garlic powder, and onion powder to create a batter.

3. Dip each cauliflower floret into the batter, ensuring they are well coated, and place them on the prepared baking sheet.

4. Bake in the oven for 20-25 minutes until the cauliflower is crispy and golden.

5. Toss the baked cauliflower in buffalo sauce until evenly coated.

6. Serve with vegan ranch dressing and celery sticks on the side.

Benefits:

These cauliflower buffalo wings are a healthier alternative to traditional chicken wings. They are rich in vitamins and minerals from cauliflower and almond flour. They support bone health, immune function, and are a delicious party snack.

Recipe 15: Vegan Avocado and Chickpea Salad Sandwich

Ingredients:

- 1 can chickpeas, drained and rinsed
- 1 ripe avocado, mashed
- 1/4 cup diced red onion
- 1/4 cup diced celery
- 2 tbsp vegan mayonnaise
- 1 tbsp Dijon mustard
- Salt and pepper to taste
- Sliced bread or whole-grain wraps
- Lettuce and sliced tomatoes for topping

Instructions:

1. In a large bowl, mash the chickpeas with a fork or potato masher until slightly chunky.

2. Add the mashed avocado, diced red onion, diced celery, vegan mayonnaise, Dijon mustard, salt, and pepper. Mix until well combined.

3. Spread the avocado and chickpea mixture onto slices of bread or wraps.

4. Top with lettuce and sliced tomatoes, then close the sandwich or roll up the wrap.

Benefits:

This creamy and filling sandwich is an excellent source of plant-based protein, healthy fats, and fiber. It supports brain health, provides sustained energy, and is a great option for a quick lunch.

Recipe 16: Vegan Coconut Curry Lentil Soup

Ingredients:

- 1 cup red lentils
- 1 can coconut milk
- 1 cup diced potatoes
- 1 cup diced carrots
- 1 cup chopped spinach
- 1 small onion, diced
- 2 cloves garlic, minced
- 1 tbsp curry powder
- 1 tsp ground turmeric
- 4 cups vegetable broth
- 1 tbsp coconut oil
- Fresh cilantro for garnish

Instructions:

1. In a large pot, heat coconut oil over medium heat.

2. Add diced onions and minced garlic, sauté until softened.

3. Stir in the curry powder and ground turmeric, toasting the spices for a minute.

4. Add the red lentils, diced potatoes, and diced carrots, stirring to coat them in the spices.

5. Pour in the vegetable broth and bring to a simmer. Cook for about 15-20 minutes or until the lentils and vegetables are tender.

6. Stir in the coconut milk and chopped spinach, allowing the soup to heat through.

7. Serve hot, garnished with fresh cilantro.

Benefits:

This creamy and aromatic soup is a fantastic source of plant-based protein, fiber, and healthy fats from coconut milk. It supports immune function, aids digestion, and is a comforting meal.

Recipe 17: Vegan Spinach and Mushroom Stuffed Shells

Ingredients:

- 1 box jumbo pasta shells (about 20 shells)
- 1 cup chopped spinach
- 1 cup sliced mushrooms
- 1 cup diced tomatoes (canned or fresh)
- 1 cup vegan ricotta cheese (store-bought or homemade)
- 1/4 cup nutritional yeast
- 1 tsp dried basil
- 1 tsp dried oregano
- Salt and pepper to taste
- 2 cups marinara sauce

Instructions:

1. Preheat the oven to 375°F (190°C). Cook the jumbo pasta shells according to package instructions, then drain and set aside.

2. In a large skillet, sauté chopped spinach, sliced mushrooms, and diced tomatoes until the vegetables are softened.

3. In a bowl, mix together the sautéed vegetables, vegan ricotta cheese, nutritional yeast, dried basil, dried oregano, salt, and pepper.

4. Stuff each cooked pasta shell with the vegetable and cheese mixture.

5. Spread a thin layer of marinara sauce in a baking dish and arrange the stuffed shells on top.

6. Cover the shells with the remaining marinara sauce.

7. Bake in the oven for 20-25 minutes until heated through and bubbly.

Benefits:

These stuffed shells are a delicious and nutritious pasta dish, providing a combination of vitamins and minerals from spinach, mushrooms, and tomatoes. They support bone health, contribute to a balanced diet, and make a delightful dinner option.

Recipe 18: Vegan Teriyaki Tofu Skewers

Ingredients:

- 1 block of firm tofu, cubed

- 1 cup sliced bell peppers

- 1 cup sliced zucchini

- 1 cup pineapple chunks

- 1/4 cup soy sauce

- 2 tbsp maple syrup

- 1 tbsp rice vinegar
- 1 tbsp sesame oil
- 1 tsp grated ginger
- Wooden skewers, soaked in water

Instructions:

1. In a bowl, whisk together soy sauce, maple syrup, rice vinegar, sesame oil, and grated ginger to create the teriyaki marinade.

2. Marinate the cubed tofu in the teriyaki sauce for at least 30 minutes or longer.

3. Preheat the grill or grill pan over medium-high heat.

4. Thread the marinated tofu, sliced bell peppers, zucchini, and pineapple chunks onto the soaked wooden skewers.

5. Grill the skewers for 3-4 minutes on each side or until the tofu is lightly charred and the vegetables are tender.

6. Serve the teriyaki tofu skewers over cooked rice, drizzling any remaining marinade as a sauce.

Benefits:

These flavorful skewers are a great source of plant-based protein, antioxidants, and fiber from the tofu and vegetables. They support muscle health, provide sustained energy, and are perfect for summer grilling.

Recipe 19: Vegan Chocolate Chia Pudding

Ingredients:

- 1/4 cup chia seeds

- 1 cup plant-based milk (such as almond or coconut milk)

- 2 tbsp cocoa powder

- 2 tbsp maple syrup

- 1/2 tsp vanilla extract

- Fresh berries for topping

Instructions:

1. In a jar or bowl, combine chia seeds, plant-based milk, cocoa powder, maple syrup, and vanilla extract.

2. Stir well to ensure the chia seeds are evenly distributed.

3. Cover the jar or bowl and refrigerate for at least 2 hours or overnight, allowing the chia seeds to absorb the liquid and create a pudding-like texture.

4. Stir the chia pudding before serving and top with fresh berries.

Benefits:

This indulgent dessert is a nutritious treat, offering omega-3 fatty acids from chia seeds and antioxidants from cocoa powder. It supports brain health, provides a guilt-free sweet treat, and is an excellent alternative to traditional pudding.

Recipe 20: Vegan Mediterranean Couscous Salad

Ingredients:

- 1 cup cooked couscous
- 1 cup chopped cucumber
- 1 cup cherry tomatoes, halved
- 1/2 cup chopped red onion
- 1/4 cup chopped Kalamata olives
- 1/4 cup crumbled vegan feta cheese
- 2 tbsp extra-virgin olive oil
- 1 tbsp lemon juice
- 1 tsp dried oregano
- Salt and pepper to taste
- Fresh parsley for garnish

Instructions:

1. In a large bowl, combine cooked couscous, chopped cucumber, cherry tomatoes, red onion, Kalamata olives, and vegan feta cheese.

2. In a separate small bowl, whisk together extra-virgin olive oil, lemon juice, dried oregano, salt, and pepper to make the dressing.

3. Pour the dressing over the couscous salad and toss to combine.

4. Garnish with fresh parsley before serving.

Benefits:

This refreshing and light salad is a great source of whole grains, healthy fats, and antioxidants. It supports heart health, provides sustained energy, and makes for a delightful side dish.

CONCLUSION

As we come to the end of this culinary adventure, we hope that these Fast, Cheap, and Delicious Vegan recipes have brought joy and inspiration to your kitchen. Embracing a plant-based lifestyle doesn't mean sacrificing flavor, variety, or convenience. On the contrary, it opens up a world of possibilities, where fresh ingredients and creative combinations can take center stage in every meal.

Throughout this collection, we've witnessed the incredible potential of vegan cuisine, not just in its delectable taste but also in its positive impact on our health and the environment. These recipes have shown us that with a little imagination and the right ingredients, we can create dishes that nourish our bodies and delight our taste buds, all while being mindful of our budgets and time constraints.

We hope these recipes have empowered you to explore the vast world of vegan cooking further, encouraging you to experiment with your own twists and additions. Whether you're a seasoned vegan or new to the plant-based journey, our hope is that these recipes have opened your eyes to the endless possibilities and deliciousness that await in the world of vegan cuisine.

As you continue to enjoy these dishes and embark on your own culinary endeavors, remember that food is not just nourishment for the body but also a celebration of life and the moments we share with loved ones. May these recipes not only inspire you to create delightful meals but also to savor every bite, appreciating the beauty of nourishing ourselves and the planet in harmony.

Thank you for joining us on this flavorful journey, and remember, the adventure doesn't end here. There are countless more ingredients to explore, combinations to try, and tastes to savor. Happy cooking, happy eating, and here's to a joyful and delicious vegan lifestyle!